BROWN RICE SYRUP

ALL YOU SHOULD KNOW ABOUT BROWN RICE SYRUP

TERRANCE B. WITNEY

Table of Contents

CHAPTER ONE

What Is Brown Rice Syrup?

Brown rice syrup is a liquid sugar alternative that is gluten-free, vegan, and comes from brown rice. Asia, Europe, and the United States are the essential locations the place it is made. A sweetener made from brown rice is referred to as brown rice syrup. It has lengthy records of use in Asian delicacies and is turning into increasingly more famous amongst human beings searching for a plant-based choice to sophisticated sugar. This syrup can be used as-is or in baking and cooking to sweeten ingredients with fewer calories. However, it ought to be substituted for in recipes in order to work properly.

How Does Brown Rice Syrup Work?

Maltose syrup, rice syrup, and rice malt syrup are different names for brown rice syrup. Brown rice is cooked and uncovered to herbal enzymes to make it. These spoil down and convert the starches in the rice into sugars (maltose, maltotriose, and glucose), which are then decreased to a mild brown syrup with the aid of boiling.

The syrup regularly consists of natural ingredients. It has excessive glycemic index, low stages of glucose, and consists of no gluten or fructose. It can also be desired with the aid of vegans to subtle sugar, which is now and again sophisticated the use of animal bone char. Rice milk and processed meals that are marketed as herbal and healthy, like granola bars and beverages, which would in any other case be made with subtle sugars or excessive fructose corn syrup (HFCS), often encompass it in their formulations. Corn Syrup vs. Brown Rice Syrup In recipes, brown rice syrup and corn syrup are regularly used interchangeably. Similar to how corn syrup has been used for a lengthy time in the United States, brown rice syrup is greater normally used in Asian nations due to the availability of the meals crop. Both are glucose syrups, and their outcomes on meals and consistency are comparable. Brown rice syrup is a desirable choice to corn syrup that can be used to make sweet or for different high-temperature cooking. However, not like corn syrup, it does have a nutty flavor.

The software of brown rice syrup is similar to that of any different liquid sweetener. For a little greater sweetness, use it in drinks like espresso and tea or in any recipe that calls for a liquid sweetener. Similar to maple syrup, it can additionally be drizzled over waffles and pancakes. It can additionally be used as an ice cream or dessert topping for some people.

CHAPTER TWO
How to Cook with Brown Rice Syrup

Brown rice syrup can be used straight out of the jar and does no longer require any extra preparation. It works properly as a liquid sweetener in cooked and uncooked foods, specifically if you desire to decrease the quantity of sugar in a recipe or make it vegan or gluten-free. It can make baked items too crispy when used in baking. In some recipes, it can be mixed with any other liquid sweetener to repair this. What's the taste like? A lot much less candy than agave nectar, honey, and sugar is brown rice syrup. The flavor is a little bit nutty, however some people say it tastes like butterscotch.

Substitutes for Brown Rice Syrup

Because it isn't always as candy as different liquid sweeteners, you will want to make changes when the usage of brown rice syrup in recipes. Brown rice syrup can generally be substituted for corn syrup in a 1:1 ratio.

The distinction with different sweeteners is typically 1/4 cup, however this can be modified to swimsuit your taste. For instance, you can alternative 3/4 cup of honey, barley malt syrup, or maple syrup for the 1 cup of brown rice syrup known as for in a recipe. The ratio of 3/4 cup white granulated sugar to 1 cup brown rice syrup is the same; however, switching from a liquid to a dry sweetener can alter the food's consistency. When changing 1 cup of brown rice syrup, use solely half of cup of molasses due to the fact it has a improved flavor. For every cup of brown rice syrup, solely three tablespoons of date syrup are required.

Recipes Using Brown Rice Syrup Since brown rice syrup is vegan, it is regularly used in vegan-friendly dishes. It can additionally be used to sweeten recipes in location of honey

Where to Buy Brown Rice Syrup

This syrup is one of the extra high-priced liquid sweeteners available. It is handy online, in Asian markets, and in natural-food-focused distinctiveness grocery stores. It can be observed in the baking part alongside different sweeteners. The majority of brown rice syrup can be saved except being refrigerated, even though doing so can make it

closing longer. It will maintain nicely for up to a yr at room temperature as soon as it is opened. If the syrup crystallizes in the jar, like with honey, stir it in heat water to dissolve the crystals. The whole jar needs to be thrown out if you are aware of any mould   growing.
The big difference between what's suitable for you and what's terrible for you can get simply tough to make in the sugary, swirling world. One of the many sugar substitutes out there is brown rice syrup, and given that it consists of brown rice, you would suppose it would be healthy, right? I'm right here to reply the critical questions   about   this   sugar substitute.It is made with the aid of filtering out impurities and exposing cooked rice to enzymes that destroy down starches into smaller sugars. A thick, candy syrup is the stop result.

CHAPTER THREE

How Does Brown Rice Syrup Work?

Maltotriose (52 percent), maltose (45 percent), and glucose (3%) are the three sugars in brown rice syrup. However, the names must now not deceive you. Maltotriose has three glucose molecules, whereas maltose solely has two. As a result, the physique makes use of brown rice syrup like one hundred percent glucose. Brown rice syrup, additionally recognised as rice syrup or rice malt syrup, is a sweetener made from brown rice. Brown rice is fermented, the starches are damaged down through enzymes, and the combination is decreased till it has the consistency of syrup. Brown rice syrup is if truth be told simply glucose when damaged down. As a choice to white sugar, high-fructose corn syrup, and synthetic sweeteners, you can locate brown rice syrup in many natural and fitness meals products, like breakfast cereal and snack bars. Brown rice syrup is additionally used in some recipes, like these for granola bars. Is it a healthful choice to sugar? Despite the reality that brown rice syrup can be discovered in a lot of natural and fitness meals products, there are no inherent benefits to the use of brown rice syrup over different sugar alternatives. According to researchers, "Even though brown rice syrup is promoted as plant-based, gluten-free, and normally 'healthy,' in the end, it is damaged down into easy sugars in our bodies, simply like ordinary white sugar and high-fructose corn syrup."

According to some studies, brown rice syrup has a greater glycemic index, which shows that the sugar is absorbed extra rapidly and motives a spike in blood sugar levels.

What is the GI?

The GI also known as the glycemic index of brown rice syrup, The glycemic index, or GI, is a metric that shows how rapidly a meals can increase blood sugar. Which measures how rapidly your physique converts sugar into glucose, is a whopping ninety eight out of a hundred Out of all the processed sugars, along with white sugar and high-fructose corn syrup, is a metric that shows how rapidly a meals can increase blood sugar? it has the easiest GI. Foods with a excessive glycemic index, such as bread, puffed wheat cereals, crackers, and different snacks, are shortly absorbed into the bloodstream and purpose fast adjustments in blood level. Because you sense fuller for a shorter duration of time, This is proof to endorse that consuming a lot of meals with a excessive glycemic index might also lead to weight problems When you eat meals with a excessive GI, your blood sugar and insulin degrees skyrocket earlier than plummeting, ensuing in starvation and cravings. The GI database maintained shows that rice syrup has an extraordinarily excessive glycemic index of ninety eight. It has a GI of 60–70, which is notably greater than that of desk sugar and almost each and every different reachable sweetener.

Rice syrup has a glycemic index of 98, which is greater than nearly each different sweetener on the market. If you consume it, it is very probable to reason speedy spikes in blood sugar

CHAPTER FOUR

Nutrient Contents and Compositions

Brown rice syrup, additionally acknowledged as rice malt syrup or genuinely rice syrup, is mainly composed of glucose. However, you may marvel if it is higher for you than different sweeteners.

You will research whether or not brown rice syrup is really helpful to your fitness in this article. Brown rice syrup is made by means of changing the starch in cooked rice into sugars that are effortless to digest. Nutrient Content Although brown rice syrup is very low in nutrients, it is extraordinarily nutritious.

It may additionally incorporate a small quantity of minerals like calcium and potassium, however in contrast to entire foods, these quantities are negligible. Remember that this syrup has a lot of sugar.

As a result, brown rice syrup has a lot of energy however few vital nutrients. Glucose versus fructose there is a lot of debate about why introduced sugar is awful for you. Some persons accept as true with it is virtually due to the reality that it lacks simply all nutritional vitamins and minerals, making it doubtlessly unsafe to your teeth. But there is proof that its fructose is mainly harmful.

Obviously, fructose does now not drastically elevate blood sugar tiers like glucose does. Consequently, it is higher for diabetics. However, whilst fructose can be metabolized in full-size portions with the aid of your liver, glucose can be metabolized through any telephone in your physique. Excessive fructose consumption can also be one of the underlying motives of two kind diabetes, in accordance to some scientists. Insulin resistance, fatty liver, and increased triglyceride degrees have all been linked to ingesting a lot of fructose

since glucose can be metabolized with the aid of each and every phone in your body, it should not have an effect on liver feature in the equal way.

Penalties of ingesting brown rice syrup

Additionally, the penalties of ingesting brown rice syrup are that High-fructose corn syrup is often substituted for brown rice syrup in processed foods. In addition to ingesting an immoderate quantity of calories, brought sugars like brown rice syrup can also purpose weight achieve and ailments like diabetes and coronary heart disease. One of the worst matters about the cutting-edge eating regimen is the introduced sugar.

It is composed of glucose and fructose, two easy sugars. While a small quantity of fructose from fruit is fine, a lot of fructose from introduced sugar might also be horrific for your fitness. Because of this, many persons use low-fructose sweeteners like brown rice syrup rather than that of fructose.

High quality factor of brown rice syrup

The solely high quality factor of brown rice syrup is its excessive glucose content. Keep in idea that fruits, which are nutritious foods, do no longer fall below any of this. Brown rice syrup does no longer incorporate fructose, so it ought to now not have the equal bad consequences on liver characteristic and metabolic fitness as normal sugar. However, they do incorporate a lot of nutrients, fiber, and different nutrients.

CHAPTER FIVE

Content of Arsenic

Arsenic is a toxic chemical that regularly exists in hint quantities in some foods, such as rice and rice syrup.

Organic brown rice syrup's arsenic content material used to be the challenge of one study. It examined merchandise sweetened with rice syrup, such as baby formula, as nicely as remote syrups these merchandise contained a lot of arsenic, which used to be located to be a problem. Arsenic concentrations in the formulation have been 20 instances greater than these in these that have been no longer sweetened with rice syrup.

However, in accordance to the Food and Drug Administration (FDA), these quantities are inadequate to pose a risk.

However, brown rice syrup-sweetened baby formulation is possibly nice averted entirely. Rice syrups and merchandise sweetened with them have been discovered to comprise sizeable quantities of arsenic. This has the practicable to be worrying. High fructose corn syrup has been changed through natural brown rice syrup as a sweetener in many ingredients that are marketed as "natural" or "healthy." Enzymes are used to destroy down the starch in cooked whole-grain rice into the sugars maltose, maltotriose, and a small quantity of glucose. The candy liquid is strained and boiled down into syrup. Organic brown rice syrup is appropriate for vegan diets and does no longer comprise gluten. in contrast to forty two for desk sugar.

Organic brown rice sugar can be observed in a range of foods, together with cereal bars, power drinks, and child milk formula. Arsenic is, in fact, the hassle with natural brown rice formula's safety. Arsenic tiers in child formula, cereal, power bars, and high-energy drinks used with the aid of patience athletes had been substantially greater than the EPA's 2001 restriction of 10 components per billion (ppb) for public ingesting water, in accordance to a Dartmouth University find out about posted in 2012. Cereal bars containing natural brown rice syrup had concentrations ranging from 23 to 128 ppb; One power drink had eighty four components per billion (ppb) and two had 171 ppb.

A soy-based method had 21.4 ppb, whilst the dairy child system had 8.6 ppb.

Rice Flora

Rice itself is the supply of the arsenic, and brown rice includes greater of it than white rice. Rice flora have a tendency to soak up arsenic greater with ease than different meals crops, no matter the truth that arsenic is naturally current in soil and water. Researchers say that this occurs regardless of whether or not natural or traditional rice plant lives are grown. The researchers additionally say that it does not comprehend of any statistics that says natural rice has greater arsenic than traditional rice.

Long-term publicity to excessive stages of arsenic is linked to greater costs of coronary heart ailment as properly as skin, bladder, and lung cancers, even although the mechanism by means of which arsenic builds up in the physique is now not totally clear. It's viable that kids who eat too a great deal meals containing arsenic will have a decrease IQ and be much less in a position to assume critically. However, it is unknown whether or not small quantities of arsenic amassed over time from rice and different meals will have long-term fitness effects. The researchers pointed out that preceding lookup hasn't seemed at arsenic publicity in youth at stages same to these in the child formulation they tested. They say to use formulation that do not have brown rice syrup in them. According to the researchers, ingesting two to three massive servings of cereal or power bars every day may want to add 10 ppb of inorganic arsenic to your diet. If you discover yourself in want of electricity or diet bars, I suggest going with ones that have no delivered sugars at all and are sweetened with whole, dried fruit.

www.ingramcontent.com/pod-product-compliance
Lightning Source LLC
Chambersburg PA
CBHW070946250726
48663CB00001B/91